75

DAY

A Tactical Guide To Winning the War With Yourself.

Andy Friend

Copyright © 2023 by Andry Friend

This book is a work of fiction. Any resemblance to actual events, locales, or persons, living or dead, is entirely coincidental.

Published by Smart Service Press

Paperback ISBN: 9789693192872

Printed in the United States of America

Cover design by BC GRAHAM

Editor and Illustrator: Elsie Bloomfield

Download Free Now!

75
HARD

A TACTICAL GUIDE TO WINNING
THE WAR WITH YOURSELF

A JOURNAL

SCAN THIS
CODE TO GET
THIS BOOK
FREE NOW

Introduction

In an ever-changing world of uncertainties, chaos, and seemingly insurmountable challenges, one trait that sets the resilient apart from the rest is mental toughness. It is a characteristic that empowers us to confront adversity with courage, handle pressure with ease, and navigate through the stormy waters of life without faltering. "Developing Mental Toughness using a 75-Day Challenge" is an insightful guide designed to help you unlock and nurture this power within yourself.

But what exactly is mental toughness? It is the capacity to deal with obstacles, stay focused under pressure, and bounce back from failures. It involves a powerful mix of resilience, focus, determination, and emotional intelligence. Mental toughness, like any other skill, can be developed, cultivated, and fine-tuned.

This book offers you a practical, step-by-step framework designed to foster and reinforce mental toughness over a 75-day period. This approach was carefully crafted based on psychological research, neuroscience, and real-life experiences from those who have demonstrated immense mental strength in the face of adversity. Whether you are a student, athlete, professional, entrepreneur, or anyone who aims to elevate their mental strength, this book is for you.

You may wonder, "Why 75 days? Our brains are wired to resist sudden changes in behavior and lifestyle. However, research has shown that it takes approximately 66 days to form a new habit, while additional days solidify and deepen the change. By dedicating 75 days to this challenge, you not only form new habits but also allow these habits to become an integral part of your identity.

The contents of this book have been carefully chosen to address key aspects of mental toughness, such as stress resilience, emotional regulation, determination, self-discipline, and a growth mindset. As you proceed through the chapters, you will learn how to identify and face your fears, how to set goals, how to be accountable, how to overcome obstacles, how to develop a routine that fosters resilience, how to maintain focus despite distractions, and how to embrace failure as a stepping stone to success.

This book is not just about knowledge; it's about action. Each chapter provides practical exercises, strategies, and tools that can be immediately applied in daily life. By following this 75-day challenge, you are committing to a transformative journey of self-discovery, personal growth, and enhanced mental strength.

Our goal is not to help you avoid adversity or erase failure; rather, it is to equip you with the necessary skills to withstand and even grow from these experiences. With this book as your guide, you can cultivate an unshakable mindset that enables you to face any challenge with grace, confidence, and determination.

Interestingly, you will find that this 75-day challenge is not about striving for perfection or meeting some societal standard of resilience or strength. Instead, it is a personal journey towards understanding your capabilities, pushing your boundaries, and fortifying your mental and emotional resilience.

This journey might be challenging. There may be times when you feel like giving up or questioning your ability to continue. It is during these moments that your mental toughness will be tested, and it's essential to remember why you started this journey. With every hurdle you face and every setback you overcome, your mental fortitude will only become stronger, helping you shape a resilient and empowered mindset.

Throughout this book, you'll discover stories of individuals from diverse backgrounds who embarked on similar journeys to develop mental toughness. Their experiences serve as powerful testimonies to the transformative power of resilience and mental strength. These real-life stories provide a sense of relatability, motivation, and a tangible representation of the concepts we will explore.

By committing to this 75-day challenge, you are choosing to take the driver's seat in your life. You are deciding to become resilient in the face of adversity, to remain unwavering in the face of challenges, and to become the best version of yourself.

Let's begin this extraordinary journey towards mental resilience and personal mastery. Welcome to the 75-Day Challenge for developing mental toughness. This book is your first step on this transformative journey. Let's begin this challenge and awaken the mental warrior within you!

Table of Contents

How to Use This Book

First and foremost, I want to express my heartfelt gratitude for choosing this book. Your decision to invest in yourself and your mental toughness is commendable. With your dedication, this book can serve as a significant tool in your journey towards personal growth and resilience.

Now, let's dive into how you can make the most of your decision:

1. **Fully embrace the 75-Day Challenge**: You've already taken the first step by purchasing this book. Now, commit yourself to sticking with it for the full 75 days. Remember, consistency is key here, even more than intensity.

2. **Engage Actively**: This isn't a book meant for a one-time read; it's a guide for your journey. Engage with the material, scribble in the margins, and underline things that resonate

with you. Don't just read; absorb, reflect, and internalize.

3. **Do the Exercises**: Every chapter will have practical exercises. They might challenge you, but remember, that's how growth happens. The real magic happens when you step out of your comfort zone and apply what you've learned.

4. **Practice patience and compassion.** This journey isn't about becoming perfect; it's about growth and progress. There will be ups and downs. Be patient with yourself and practice self-compassion. Each setback is an opportunity to build mental toughness.

5. **Apply Your Learning**: Try to apply the principles and techniques in your daily life. Remember, the objective is to make a real, tangible difference in your life, not just learning theories.

6. **Reflect and revisit**: Make time for reflection. Pause, assess your progress, and go back to previous chapters if needed. This book is your companion for the next 75 days (and beyond).

7. **Share Your Journey**: If you're comfortable, share your journey with a trusted friend or loved one. They can be your sounding board, your cheerleader, and even your gentle reminder when things get tough.

8. **Celebrate Your Progress**: Each step you take in this journey, no matter how small, is a win. Celebrate these wins. Acknowledging your progress will fuel your motivation and solidify your commitment.

Again, thank you for picking up this book and embarking on this journey towards building mental toughness. Remember, you are not alone on this journey. I am with you, cheering you on every step of the way. Let's embark on this incredible journey together!

Chapter 1: Mental Toughness Mindset

Understanding and developing a mental toughness mindset is the bedrock of becoming mentally strong. This mindset shapes our perception of reality, dictates how we respond to adversity, and greatly influences our level of resilience and determination. Before delving deeper into the concept, let's establish one key fact: mental toughness is not about denying emotions or maintaining a facade of invulnerability. It's about demonstrating emotional intelligence, remaining composed during adversity, and showing an unfaltering will to surmount challenges.

Moreover, it's about recognizing that failure isn't a setback but an opportunity to take a different path towards success. This mindset implies that while life will present challenges and setbacks, our interpretation and response to these trials will determine our path and ultimate outcomes. It's about viewing hurdles as stepping stones rather than blockades. Importantly, this mindset isn't a birthright; it's a skill that can be fostered and honed, which is precisely what this chapter aims to help you achieve.

Resilience, confidence, focus, grit, and positivity are just a few characteristics of the mindset of mentally tough people.

1. **Resilience** is the capacity to rebound from setbacks, adjust, and persist in the face of adversity.

2. **Confidence** is their conviction in their abilities to handle whatever life throws at them.

3. **Focus** is the ability to maintain concentration and stay on task, irrespective of distractions or difficulties.

4. **Grit** is the determination to persistently work towards one's long-term goals despite obstacles and setbacks.

5. **Positivity** is the capability to sustain a positive outlook, even in testing circumstances, and engage in positive self-talk.

To cultivate a mental toughness mindset, it is crucial to nurture these traits within yourself. Here's how you can do this:

1. **Embrace Challenges**: Regard challenges as growth opportunities. Every difficulty you encounter is a potential learning and self-improvement avenue.

2. **Practice resilience**: When you face setbacks, focus on solutions rather than dwelling on the problems, extracting lessons from the experience.

3. **Believe in yourself.** Bolster confidence in your abilities. Recognize your strengths and accept your weaknesses. This belief system fortifies mental toughness, enabling you to confront challenges head-on.

4. **Maintain Focus**: Cultivate mindfulness and hone your ability to concentrate on the task at hand, regardless of distractions and complications.

5. **Develop grit**: Commit to your goals, even when progress seems sluggish or obstacles seem daunting.

6. **Cultivate positivity**: Foster a positive attitude and engage in positive self-talk.

The role of positivity in mental toughness is particularly noteworthy. A positive attitude helps to counteract stress, overcome challenges, and improve overall performance. To cultivate positivity, begin by practicing gratitude. Take note of the good things in your life, no matter how small. Engage in positive self-talk and counter negative thoughts with positive ones. Surround yourself with positive influences—people who inspire and uplift you. And remember to celebrate your victories, whether big or small.

Cultivating a mental toughness mindset is a journey, not a destination. It requires patience, practice, and persistence. Be patient with yourself, savor each step forward, and remember that every setback is a new opportunity for growth and learning.

Cultivating a positive attitude is integral to the development of mental toughness. This mindset doesn't just help you see the brighter side of things; it fundamentally changes the way you approach challenges, fostering resilience and encouraging a solution-oriented approach. Here are some practical strategies to help foster a positive attitude:

1. **Practice Gratitude**: Make it a habit to recognize and appreciate the good in your life. This could be as simple as writing down three things you're grateful for at the end of each day. Over time, this helps shift your focus from negative aspects to positive ones, enhancing overall positivity.

2. **Positive Affirmations**: Utilize positive affirmations daily to reinforce positive thinking and self-belief. These are uplifting statements you say to yourself, such as "I am capable," "I am strong," or "I can overcome this challenge." These affirmations can help shape a more positive outlook over time.

3. **Mindfulness and Meditation**: Engaging in mindfulness exercises or meditation can significantly enhance positivity. They help you stay present, preventing negative future predictions or past regrets from dominating your mind.

4. **Healthy Lifestyle**: A healthy body often leads to a healthier mind. Regular exercise, a balanced diet, and sufficient sleep can improve your mood, reduce stress, and boost your energy levels, promoting a more positive attitude.

5. **Positive Environment**: Surround yourself with positive influences. This includes people who inspire and uplift you, as well as

spaces that evoke calmness and positivity. Positivity can be infectious, so spending time with optimistic people can naturally influence your mindset.

6. **Learning and Growth Mindset**: Embrace the idea that challenges and setbacks are opportunities for learning and growth. This mindset fosters resilience and makes it easier to maintain positivity in the face of adversity.

7. **Limit Negative Influences**: Just as positivity can be infectious, so can negativity. Limit your exposure to negative influences, whether they're people who often see the worst in situations or media that instill fear or anxiety.

8. **Helping Others**: Altruistic acts, such as volunteering or simply helping a friend in need, can boost your mood and foster a more positive outlook.

9. **Celebrate wins**: Regardless of the size, celebrate your wins. Acknowledging your achievements can boost your confidence and promote positivity.

10. **Positive Visualization**: Visualize positive outcomes for situations you're anxious about. This can help reduce anxiety and encourage a more positive approach to challenges.

In the chapters to follow, we will delve further into the elements of mental toughness and provide a structured 75-day plan to help you develop and nurture this mindset. Your commitment and consistency will gradually uncover the transformative power of mental toughness within you.

This journey towards mental toughness begins in the mind. Your mind is an incredibly potent tool. It has the power to shape perceptions, influence responses to challenges, and chart the course of your life.

Chapter 2: Physical Fitness and Mental Toughness

The interconnectedness of physical fitness and mental toughness

Physical fitness and mental toughness share a symbiotic relationship, each amplifying the other's growth. A fit body houses a resilient mind. By challenging our physical limits, we inculcate discipline and determination, fortifying our mental strength. When we witness our physical transformation, our confidence gets a significant boost, reinforcing our belief in ourselves and our capabilities.

The Benefits of Exercise on Mental Health

Exercise isn't just about physical health; its impact on mental well-being is profound. During physical activity, our body releases endorphins (the natural mood lifters). They decrease feelings of pain, reduce stress and anxiety, and promote a sense of calm and well-being. Regular physical activity has been found to alleviate symptoms of depression and even enhance cognitive function, supporting memory and thinking skills.

Exercise is an investment in your mind-body health. As your physical health improves, you'll find a positive effect on your mood, stress levels, and even self-esteem. These benefits of exercise for mental health bolster your journey towards mental toughness.

Incorporating cardiovascular and strength training into your routine

In our 75-Day Challenge, we place strong emphasis on a balanced fitness routine. This includes both cardiovascular and strength-training exercises.

Cardiovascular exercises like jogging, cycling, swimming, or even brisk walking improve heart health, enhance lung capacity, and build stamina. These exercises also foster mental fortitude by teaching you to push past discomfort and fatigue. They challenge your willpower and resilience, contributing significantly to mental toughness.

Strength training, which includes weightlifting, resistance training, and bodyweight exercises, is equally critical. It helps in building and maintaining muscle mass, boosting metabolic health, and enhancing bone density. The discipline and consistency required in strength training instill mental resilience and determination.

While each form of exercise offers unique benefits, together they provide a balanced approach to physical fitness, ensuring all-round development and further contributing to mental toughness.

The role of hydration and nutrition in physical fitness

Physical activity alone isn't enough. Good nutrition and hydration practices must go hand in hand with it. Drinking sufficient water is crucial, especially during workouts, to replenish the fluids lost through sweat. Staying hydrated helps maintain energy levels, prevents muscle cramps, and aids overall physical performance.

Nutrition is the fuel that powers your workouts. A balanced diet, filled with lean proteins, complex carbohydrates, fruits, vegetables, and healthy fats, provides the necessary nutrients your body needs for optimum performance and recovery. Proper nutrition aids in maintaining energy levels, promoting muscle growth and repair, and supporting overall physical health.

Eating a healthy, balanced diet isn't just good for your body; it's beneficial for your brain as well. Certain foods have been linked to improved brain function, memory, and alertness, all of which contribute to mental toughness.

The Importance of Rest and Recovery

Rest is as vital as exercise in a well-rounded fitness routine. Allowing your body time to rest and recover after workouts is essential for muscle repair and strength building. It helps prevent injuries, enhances performance, and promotes growth.

Good-quality sleep is equally important. It supports various functions of the brain, including cognition, concentration, productivity, and performance. Poor sleep has been linked to mental health disorders like depression and anxiety.

As you embark on this journey, remember that while pushing your physical limits is essential, listening to your body is equally important. Embrace rest days, get enough sleep, and fuel your body with good nutrition. Physical fitness is not just about how far or fast you can go; it's about building a lifestyle that supports overall health and resilience.

In conclusion, the path to mental toughness is paved with regular exercise, balanced nutrition, adequate hydration, and restful sleep. As you go through the 75-Day Challenge, you will learn that these elements of physical fitness aren't isolated actions. They are interconnected threads woven into the fabric of a healthier, more resilient you.

Each drop of sweat shed during a strenuous workout, each nutritious meal savored, each glass of water enjoyed, and each restful night of sleep are steps closer to developing the mental toughness you seek. Embrace these elements as part of your lifestyle, not just for the challenge but as sustainable habits beyond these 75 days.

James Gordon said, "The road to mental toughness isn't easy, but remember, it's not that some people have willpower and some don't. It's that some people are ready to change and others are not." With this program, you are equipping yourself with the tools to effect that change.

This chapter sets the stage for an intricate dance between physical fitness and mental toughness, a symbiosis where each fuels the other's growth. Through the 75-Day Challenge, you will witness firsthand the transformative power of physical fitness on your mind. You will develop a deeper understanding of your capabilities, resilience, and inner strength. Embrace the process, celebrate your progress, and remember that each day is a step closer to a stronger, more resilient you.

Chapter 3: Mental Fitness and the 75-Day Program

Much like physical fitness, mental fitness is an essential aspect of overall well-being, performance, and resilience. It refers to our cognitive and emotional health, enabling us to handle stress, overcome challenges, maintain focus, and engage with the world positively and productively. Developing mental fitness requires practice, just like building physical strength, and this chapter is designed to provide a roadmap for strengthening your mental muscles through a strategic 75-day program.

Understanding Mental Fitness

At its core, mental fitness is about strengthening our minds' resilience, flexibility, and efficiency. It's about training our brains to effectively handle life's ups and downs and bounce back from adversity. It involves cultivating habits that enhance cognitive functioning, emotional well-being, and mental resilience.

Importance of Mental Fitness Exercises

Mental fitness exercises like mindfulness, meditation, and cognitive workouts are tools to enhance our mental strength. They provide us with the ability to focus, manage our emotions, and think clearly under pressure.

1. *Mindfulness:* Mindfulness teaches us to live in the present moment, helping us reduce anxiety, improve focus, and manage stress effectively. It allows us to acknowledge our thoughts and emotions without judgment, allowing us to respond rather than react to challenging situations.

2. *Meditation:* Meditation is a technique that encourages mental clarity and emotional calmness. Regular meditation practice can enhance self-awareness, promote relaxation, reduce stress, and increase mental resilience. It can help us cultivate a sense of inner peace that bolsters our mental strength.

3. **Cognitive Workouts:** Cognitive workouts involve engaging in activities that challenge the brain, such as puzzles, reading, writing, or learning a new skill. These exercises stimulate the brain, improving cognitive flexibility, memory, focus, and creativity.

The 75-Day Mental Fitness Program

This program is designed to be an incremental journey, gradually increasing the intensity and complexity of mental fitness exercises over 75 days. It's built on the premise that mental toughness, much like physical strength, takes time and consistent effort to develop. Here's a brief outline of the structure:

- **Weeks 1-3 (Building Foundations):** These weeks introduce the basics of mindfulness, meditation, and cognitive exercises. You'll start with shorter exercises, gradually building your mental endurance.

In these initial weeks, you're just getting started. You'll spend 10 minutes each day practicing mindfulness, starting with simple activities like mindful eating or mindful walking. This could be as simple as noticing the sensation of your feet hitting the ground or savoring each bite of your meal.

At the same time, you'll begin to incorporate basic meditation into your routine. Start with 5 minutes of deep breathing meditation each day, focusing on your breath and letting go of any intrusive thoughts.

For cognitive exercises, spend 15 minutes each day on a brain-boosting activity. This could be solving a crossword puzzle, reading a challenging book, or learning a new skill, like a foreign language or a musical instrument.

- **Weeks 4-6 (Increasing Intensity):** As you become more comfortable with these exercises, the program intensifies. You'll be challenged to dig deeper into your mental strength, pushing your mental boundaries.

Now that you've laid the foundation, it's time to increase the intensity. Bump your daily mindfulness practice up to 20 minutes, perhaps incorporating mindful listening —tuning into and focusing on the sounds around you.

Your daily meditation should also increase to 10 minutes. You can try guided meditations focusing on body awareness or loving-kindness. Increase your cognitive workouts to 30 minutes a day. This could involve more complex puzzles, engaging with educational material, or progressing in your new skill.

- *Weeks 7-9 (Mastering Techniques):* This phase focuses on refining and mastering these techniques. You'll start integrating these practices into your daily routine.

In this phase, your mindfulness practice should become a part of your daily life. Try to bring mindfulness into regular activities, like brushing your teeth, doing the dishes, or even during work tasks.

Increase your meditation time to 15 minutes per day. Consider exploring different types of meditation, such as mantra meditation or mindfulness meditation.

For your cognitive workouts, focus on mastery. Choose one cognitive activity you particularly enjoy and dedicate your cognitive workout time to progressing in this area.

- **Weeks 10–11 (Consolidation and Expansion):** In the final weeks, you'll consolidate your skills and explore new ways to apply your mental toughness.

In the final weeks, you're consolidating your mental fitness habits and challenging yourself to expand your boundaries. Try to incorporate mindfulness into even more aspects of your daily life, making it an almost constant practice.

Your daily meditation should now be 20 minutes. You might consider trying meditative practices that incorporate movement, such as yoga or tai chi.

With your cognitive workouts, continue to challenge yourself. This could mean tackling a particularly difficult puzzle or pushing yourself to a new level in a cognitive skill you've been developing.

Remember, the goal of this program isn't to become perfect at mindfulness, meditation, or cognitive exercises. It's about building mental toughness, resilience, and adaptability. Some days will be harder than others, and that's okay. The key is to keep pushing forward, continue practicing, and maintain a positive and resilient mindset.

The Connection between Physical and Mental Fitness

Physical fitness and mental fitness are intertwined. Regular physical exercise not only strengthens our bodies but also has a profound impact on our mental health. It helps manage stress, improve mood, enhance concentration, and promote better sleep. Thus, the 75-day program includes recommendations for physical activities that complement mental fitness exercises.

By following this 75-day program, you'll not only enhance your mental toughness but also foster a healthier relationship with your mind and body. You'll gain tools and techniques that will support you through life's challenges, turning obstacles into opportunities for growth and learning. Remember, developing mental toughness is a journey, not a destination, and each step you take in this 75-day challenge is a step toward a stronger, more resilient you.

Chapter 4: Goal Setting

Setting goals is like setting a course for a ship. Without a clear direction, the ship would aimlessly sail, vulnerable to the winds and currents. Similarly, without well-defined goals, our efforts may be scattered and inefficient. Thus, goal setting serves as a pivotal cornerstone in the journey of developing mental toughness.

The Importance of Setting Specific, Measurable, and Achievable Goals

Specificity in goal-setting provides a clear understanding of what we aim to accomplish. A goal like "I want to be healthier" is admirable but vague. How can we measure health? What does being healthier look like? However, a goal like "I want to be able to run 5 kilometers without stopping within the next three months" is specific, providing a clear target and timeframe.

Measurement allows us to track progress, offering tangible evidence of our advancement. It lets us know how far we have come and how far we need to go. Staying with the example above, measuring progress might include timing our runs or noting the distance we can run without stopping. This clear feedback allows us to adjust our strategies if needed and motivates us as we see ourselves getting closer to our goal.

The achievability of a goal is also essential. Setting unrealistic or overly ambitious goals can lead to frustration and demotivation. Our goals should challenge us but remain within the realm of possibility given our abilities and circumstances. It's about finding the right balance—goals should be stretching but not snapping.

Breaking down larger goals into smaller, manageable steps

Having a grand goal can be inspiring, but it can also be daunting. Breaking it down into smaller, more manageable steps makes the journey less overwhelming and more achievable. These smaller steps are like the rungs of a ladder, leading us towards our main goal.

For example, if our goal is to run a marathon, we don't start by running 42 kilometers on the first day. Instead, we break this down into smaller steps. We might start by running a couple of kilometers a day, then gradually increase the distance each week.

Each of these steps should also be specific, measurable, and achievable, serving as mini-goals that guide us towards our overall goal. By focusing on one step at a time, we can make consistent progress without feeling overwhelmed. This method also allows for small victories along the way, which serve as motivation boosters.

Staying Motivated and On Track towards Your Goals

Staying motivated and on track can often be a challenge, especially when progress is slow or obstacles arise. Here are some strategies that can help:

1. **Visualize Your Goals**: Visualization is a powerful tool that can keep us motivated. Imagine how it will feel to achieve your goal. Visualize the benefits and the sense of accomplishment. This mental picture can serve as a source of inspiration when motivation wanes.

2. **Create a Plan:** A clear plan outlines the steps needed to reach your goal. It provides structure and serves as a roadmap for your journey. Revisit and adjust your plan as necessary, and remember, it's okay to be flexible.

3. **Celebrate Progress**: Recognize and celebrate your progress, no matter how small. These celebrations can reinforce positive behavior and boost your motivation to keep going.

4. **Stay Accountable**: Share your goal with someone you trust. This could be a friend, a family member, or a mentor. They can

provide support, encouragement, and a gentle push when needed.

5. **Maintain a Positive Mindset**: Keep a positive attitude, even when faced with setbacks. View these as learning opportunities rather than failures. A positive mindset can help you stay resilient and persistent in the pursuit of your goals.

In conclusion, goal-setting is a vital step in the journey towards developing mental toughness. It gives us a clear direction and empowers us to take active control of our lives. By setting specific, measurable, and achievable goals, we create a blueprint for success.

Yet setting a goal is just the beginning. Breaking down larger goals into smaller, manageable steps helps us maintain momentum and prevent feeling overwhelmed. It provides us with a series of manageable tasks that cumulatively lead us to our ultimate goal.

Moreover, motivation plays a critical role in staying on track. Employing strategies such as visualization, celebrating progress, accountability, and maintaining a positive mindset can help us remain motivated and focused.

However, it's crucial to remember that setbacks and obstacles are an inevitable part of the journey. They aren't signs of failure, but opportunities to learn and grow. Each hurdle we overcome serves to make us tougher, both mentally and emotionally, bringing us a step closer to our goals and fostering our mental toughness.

Keep in mind that everyone's journey is unique, and there is no 'one size fits all' approach to achieving our goals. It's important to remain flexible and adjust our strategies as required, always staying true to our abilities, circumstances, and pace.

Remember, the objective isn't just to achieve our goals but to cultivate mental toughness in the process. This way, we are not only moving closer to our current goal but also equipping ourselves with the skills, mindset, and resilience to conquer future challenges.

As we close this chapter, I urge you to take a moment and reflect on your own goals. Are they specific, measurable, and achievable? Have you broken them down into smaller, manageable steps? Do you have strategies in place to stay motivated? The next time you set a goal, consider these points, for they are not only essential in achieving your goal but also in nurturing your mental toughness.

The journey to developing mental toughness is a marathon, not a sprint. Stay consistent, celebrate your progress, learn from your setbacks, and remember that every step you take, no matter how small, brings you closer to your goal and builds your mental toughness. Let's embrace this journey together and emerge stronger, one goal at a time.

Chapter 5: Accountability

Accountability, one of the most important facets of mental toughness, is a concept often underestimated in its power to drive change and growth. In the realm of mental toughness, accountability translates to owning your decisions, actions, and their outcomes, both good and bad. It also entails setting personal standards and holding yourself to them.

Benefits of Accountability on Motivation and Goal Achievement

Accountability plays a vital role in motivation and goal achievement. When we hold ourselves accountable, we create a sense of responsibility for our actions. This encourages a consistent behavior pattern aligned with our set goals. We're more likely to commit to our tasks and objectives when we know that we alone are responsible for the outcomes.

Accountability also creates a sense of ownership over our success. Every milestone achieved reinforces our belief in our capabilities, fueling motivation. Knowing that we have the power to influence our success can be incredibly empowering and serves as a significant motivating factor to push further towards our goals.

Moreover, accountability helps maintain focus on the goal. It requires regular check-ins with our progress, which keeps the goal fresh in our minds, reducing the chance of being sidetracked by distractions or lesser priorities.

Strategies for Finding Accountability Partners and Support Networks

A powerful method of fostering accountability is to have an accountability partner or join a support network. These can be friends, family members, mentors, or even professional coaches. Here are some strategies to find the right accountability partner:

1. Shared Goals or Values: Look for someone who shares similar goals or values. They'll understand your journey better and can provide relevant advice or encouragement.

2. Trust and openness: An ideal accountability partner is someone you trust and feel comfortable sharing your struggles and victories with. They need to be someone you can be honest with and who can provide constructive criticism when necessary.

3. Join a group or network: There are numerous online and offline groups centered on personal growth and mental toughness. These groups can provide a supportive environment where everyone is committed to growth.

4. Professional Guidance: If possible, consider hiring a coach or a mentor. Their experience and expertise can provide valuable insights, and they can push you to stay committed to your goals.

The Role of Self-Accountability in Mental Toughness

Self-accountability is paramount to developing mental toughness. It allows us to take control of our lives, actions, and decisions. Self-accountability means recognizing that you're the sole proprietor of your actions and their consequences. This realization leads to a sense of control and empowerment, critical components of mental toughness.

When we practice self-accountability, we start to view challenges as opportunities for growth rather than threats. This shift in perception is crucial for building resilience, a key aspect of mental toughness.

Furthermore, self-accountability encourages a growth mindset as we begin to value effort and view failures as learning opportunities rather than as indicators of inability.

Tools for Enhancing Self-Accountability

1. Self-reflection: Regular self-reflection helps us stay aware of our progress, challenges, and areas for improvement.

2. Journaling: Keeping a daily or weekly journal of your actions, thoughts, and feelings can enhance self-accountability. It provides a record of your journey, reminding you of your commitment to your goals.

3. Self-talk: Positive self-talk reinforces belief in oneself and one's capabilities, thereby increasing self-accountability.

In summary, accountability, both externally and internally, plays a vital role in the development of mental toughness. It serves as a consistent, empowering reminder that we have control over our actions and, thereby, our growth and success. By fostering a culture of accountability in our lives, we can enhance our mental toughness, thereby preparing ourselves to face life's challenges with resilience.

Building accountability habits

Building accountability is essentially a habit-forming process. Just as we develop physical muscles through consistent exercise, we can also build our 'accountability muscle' through practice. Here are some ways to do that:

1. Set clear, measurable goals: goals should be specific, measurable, achievable, relevant, and time-bound (SMART). This gives a clear picture of what success looks like and makes it easier to hold yourself accountable.

2. Break down goals: Large goals can be overwhelming. Break them down into smaller, manageable tasks. Each completed task boosts confidence and motivation, encouraging you to continue working towards the larger goal.

3. Regular check-ins: regularly assess your progress. This helps you stay on track and

adjust your strategies as necessary. Self-reflection and journaling can aid in this process.

4. Celebrate wins: Celebrate your progress, no matter how small. This reinforces positive behavior and motivates you to maintain momentum.

Accountability in the Face of Setbacks

Setbacks are inevitable on any journey. Here's where accountability truly shines in fostering mental toughness. Being accountable means acknowledging setbacks rather than ignoring them or attributing them to external factors. This leads to learning and growth, a cornerstone of mental toughness.

When faced with a setback, assess what went wrong and why. Use this as an opportunity to learn and refine your strategy. Remember, every setback is a setup for a comeback.

The Role of Accountability in the 75-Day Challenge

Throughout the 75-Day Mental Toughness Challenge, accountability will be your steadfast ally. It will keep you committed to the daily tasks and exercises, ensure that you're progressing towards your goals, and help you bounce back from any setbacks.

As you move through the challenge, your sense of accountability will likely grow, enhancing not only your mental toughness but also your overall personal growth. Remember, the goal isn't perfection but progress. Embrace every step of the journey, even the challenging ones, as an integral part of your development.

By embracing accountability, you can maximize the benefits of the 75-Day Challenge by building mental toughness and resilience that will serve you in all areas of life. In the end, developing accountability is more than just a tool for mental toughness; it's a life skill that fosters personal growth, responsibility, and success.

Chapter 6: Overcoming Obstacles

Obstacles are inevitable; they are part of life. They come in various forms, such as personal challenges, professional hurdles, physical limitations, or external factors that seem beyond our control. However, what truly matters is not the obstacle itself, but our response to it. This chapter aims to provide you with an in-depth understanding of the role obstacles play in our lives and strategies for overcoming them, thus aiding in developing mental toughness.

Benefits of Obstacles on Motivation, Goal Achievement, and Personal Development

An obstacle often presents itself as a barrier to progress, but paradoxically, it can be a catalyst for growth, change, and personal development. Here are some of the benefits:

- **Strengthens Resolve**: Facing and overcoming obstacles often reinforces our determination to achieve our goals. The challenge can make the achievement more meaningful, strengthening our resolve to succeed.

- **Promotes Problem-Solving Skills**: Obstacles force us to think creatively and develop problem-solving skills. This creativity often leads to innovation, personal growth, and goal achievement.

- **Fosters Resilience**: Overcoming obstacles builds resilience, a crucial component of mental toughness. Every challenge we face and conquer increases our confidence in our ability to handle future difficulties.

- **Provides learning opportunities**: Every obstacle offers a learning opportunity. Mistakes and failures teach us what doesn't work, helping us improve and become better individuals.

- **Enhances Self-Esteem**: Overcoming obstacles enhances self-esteem. The pride that comes from conquering a challenge improves our self-image and instills a sense of empowerment.

Strategies for problem-solving and remaining focused in hard times to overcome obstacles

Here are some strategies for overcoming obstacles:

- **Reframe Your Perspective**: See obstacles as opportunities for growth rather than roadblocks. This shift in mindset can transform your approach to the challenge.

- **Set realistic goals**: Break down your overall goal into manageable, achievable steps. Focus on one step at a time to avoid feeling overwhelmed.

- **Embrace Flexibility**: Be flexible and adaptable in your approach. If one strategy doesn't work, be open to trying another.

- **Seek Support**: Don't hesitate to seek help. Whether it's advice from a mentor, emotional support from a friend, or professional help, having a support system is crucial.

- **Practice self-care**: Take care of your physical and mental health. Practice stress-relieving activities, eat healthily, exercise regularly, and ensure you get enough rest.

The Role of Obstacles in Mental Toughness

Obstacles play a significant role in the development of mental toughness.

- **Resilience**: By challenging us, obstacles foster resilience. Each challenge we overcome builds our resilience muscle, preparing us for future difficulties.

- **Perseverance**: Obstacles test our will to persevere. This quality of staying the course, even in the face of adversity, is a cornerstone of mental toughness.

- **Adaptability**: Overcoming obstacles often requires us to adapt and adjust our strategies. This flexibility is a key component of mental toughness.

- **Self-confidence**: Every obstacle we conquer builds our confidence in our abilities, reinforcing our belief that we can face and overcome challenges.

In conclusion, obstacles are not merely hindrances but opportunities for growth and personal development. By embracing obstacles and applying strategies to overcome them, we can cultivate mental toughness, ultimately turning challenges into stepping stones towards our goals.

Self-care and mental toughness

Self-care plays a critical role in mental toughness. Despite the somewhat misleading notion that mental toughness means pushing oneself relentlessly without rest, in reality, a crucial aspect of mental toughness is knowing when to pause and take care of oneself. Here's why self-care is essential to mental toughness:

- **Maintains Physical Health**: First and foremost, taking care of our physical health is paramount. Regular exercise, healthy eating, and sufficient sleep are key components of self-care that directly impact our mental well-being. A strong, healthy body can better endure stress, bounce back from illness faster, and have more energy reserves to draw from when faced with challenges.

- **Boosts Emotional Health**: Self-care activities such as mindfulness, meditation, journaling, and therapy can improve our emotional health by reducing anxiety and depression and improving mood. Good emotional health allows us to better understand and manage our feelings, which is crucial when facing stressful situations requiring mental toughness.

- **Promotes Self-Reflection and Self-Awareness**: Self-care often involves self-reflection and introspection, which boosts self-awareness. This awareness is important for recognizing our limits, identifying what we need for our well-being, and understanding our emotional responses. This heightened self-awareness enables us to make better decisions and improve our coping strategies, thus enhancing mental toughness.

- **Prevents Burnout:** Consistent self-care can stop burnout, a condition of prolonged stress-induced emotional, physical, and mental exhaustion. It's harder to be mentally tough when you're burned out and depleted. Regular self-care ensures that we recharge and replenish our mental and physical energy, enabling us to tackle challenges with greater vigor.

- **Enhances Self-Worth and Confidence**: Engaging in self-care sends a positive message to our psyche that we matter, boosting self-esteem and confidence. A high sense of self-worth and confidence allows us to face difficulties more readily, contributing to greater mental toughness.

In essence, self-care isn't a luxury or a selfish act; it's a fundamental part of building and maintaining mental toughness. When we care for ourselves effectively, we're more able to handle stress, adapt to change, and overcome adversity—all critical aspects of mental toughness. In your journey to develop mental toughness, remember that taking time to rest and rejuvenate is as important as pushing forward and rising to challenges.

Chapter 7: Developing Resilience

Resilience is the cornerstone of mental toughness. It is the ability to bounce back from adversity, adapt to change, and keep going in the face of hardship. This trait becomes increasingly important as we face life's inevitable challenges.

Learning from setbacks and failures

Understanding the importance of learning from setbacks and failures is a significant part of developing resilience. Failure, despite its negative connotation, is an invaluable teacher. It provides us with unique learning opportunities and gives us insights into what works and what doesn't.

Each setback you encounter is a test of your resilience. How you respond to these tests determines your level of mental toughness. Those who view setbacks as an opportunity for growth and learning tend to have higher levels of resilience.

When faced with failure, instead of dwelling on the negative, ask yourself, what can I learn from this experience? What can I do differently next time? What strengths did I discover about myself in the process? Answering these questions helps change your perspective on failure, making it a stepping stone rather than an obstacle to success.

Reframing negative experiences

Reframing is a powerful psychological tool that involves changing your perspective on a challenging situation to make it more manageable or positive. It involves shifting your focus from the negative aspects of a situation to the positive ones, or the lessons that can be learned.

This does not mean ignoring reality or denying the challenge. Instead, it is about finding a silver lining, which can fuel your motivation and inspire you to overcome similar situations in the future. For example, if you didn't get the job you interviewed for, instead of viewing it as a failure, consider it a practice that has prepared you better for future interviews.

Self-reflection and self-awareness

Self-reflection and self-awareness are critical to developing resilience. They involve understanding your thoughts, emotions, and reactions to various situations. Being self-aware allows you to identify your strengths and weaknesses, understand your stressors, and recognize your response patterns.

Reflecting on your experiences can help you identify patterns in your behaviors and reactions, providing insights into what strategies work best for you in dealing with adversity. Regularly practicing self-reflection can aid in continuous self-improvement and growth, contributing to resilience.

Journaling is an excellent tool for reflection. By writing about your experiences, thoughts, and feelings, you can gain a deeper understanding of yourself, which can help you navigate through challenging situations more effectively.

Building a growth mindset

A growth mindset, a concept popularized by psychologist Carol Dweck, is the belief that abilities and intelligence can be developed over time through dedication and hard work. People with a growth mindset view challenges and setbacks as opportunities for learning and personal development.

In the context of resilience, having a growth mindset enables you to adapt to adversity and learn from your mistakes. It encourages perseverance and effort, qualities essential for overcoming obstacles and growing stronger in the process.

To cultivate a growth mindset, start by recognizing your fixed-mindset triggers. When you find yourself thinking in a fixed mindset (e.g., "I can't do this"), challenge these thoughts and replace them with growth mindset affirmations (e.g., "I can learn to do this").

Remember that resilience is a journey, not a destination. It's a skill that takes time to develop. But with persistence, self-reflection, and a willingness to learn from failures, you can build resilience and enhance your mental toughness, ready to face any challenges that come your way on your 75-day journey and beyond.

Building emotional intelligence

Emotional intelligence is another essential component in the development of resilience. It involves recognizing, understanding, and managing our emotions and the emotions of others. Emotionally intelligent individuals are better equipped to navigate stressful situations and bounce back from adversity, mainly because they can recognize and regulate their emotional responses.

Start by actively listening to your feelings. When you experience a strong emotion, instead of pushing it aside, explore it. Identify what you're feeling and why you're feeling that way. Is it a response to a recent event? A buildup of stress? Acknowledging and understanding your emotions can help you manage them more effectively.

In addition, understanding others' emotions can help you build stronger, more supportive relationships. Lean on these relationships during times of adversity. Having a solid support system can greatly enhance your resilience.

Cultivating Optimism

Optimism, a general expectation that good things will happen, is a characteristic that significantly contributes to resilience. Optimistic people are more likely to view difficulties as temporary hurdles instead of insurmountable obstacles.

Cultivating optimism starts by monitoring your internal dialogue. The way we talk to ourselves greatly affects how we view our world. Try to catch negative thoughts and reframe them into more positive ones. For instance, if you catch yourself thinking, "I'll never be able to do this," reframe it to, "This is tough, but I can work through it."

Keep in mind that cultivating optimism doesn't mean ignoring reality or glossing over problems. It's about acknowledging the reality of the situation but believing in your abilities to deal with it effectively.

Practicing Mindfulness

Mindfulness, or the practice of being fully present and engaged in the current moment, can also enhance resilience. It can help reduce stress, improve focus, and increase emotional flexibility, all of which can help you better cope with adversity.

Mindfulness can be practiced in many ways. Mindful breathing, yoga, and meditation are a few methods, but they can also be as simple as fully immersing yourself in a task or consciously paying attention to your senses.

Developing resilience is not an overnight process. It requires practice, patience, and commitment. But by learning from setbacks, reframing negative experiences, cultivating self-awareness, fostering a growth mindset, building emotional intelligence, nurturing optimism, and practicing mindfulness, you'll be well-equipped to handle life's challenges. You'll not only bounce back from adversity but also grow from it, becoming stronger and more resilient than ever before. This ability to adapt and thrive in the face of adversity is the heart of mental toughness, and it's a skill that will serve you well throughout your 75-day challenge and beyond.

Chapter 8: Mindset Shift

On the journey of personal growth and development, one of the most transformative steps you can take is shifting your mindset. The lens through which you view your experiences, capabilities, and potential profoundly influences your actions, reactions, and ultimately your life's trajectory. This chapter delves into the essential tasks of cultivating a growth mindset, developing a positive attitude, embracing self-reflection and self-awareness, and harnessing the power of gratitude. All these facets intertwine to enable a significant shift in mindset, a vital step in developing mental toughness.

Cultivating a growth mindset

A growth mindset, a term coined by psychologist Carol Dweck, is the belief that skills and abilities can be developed over time through effort, persistence, and the right strategies. This is in contrast to a fixed mindset, which believes that our abilities are innate and unchangeable.

A growth mindset is paramount to developing mental toughness because it positions challenges and failures not as insurmountable roadblocks but as opportunities for learning and growth. With a growth mindset, you understand that your potential is not predetermined; it's cultivated.

Strategies for cultivating a growth mindset include:

- **Embrace Challenges**: Seek out opportunities to push your boundaries and learn new things, understanding that discomfort often accompanies growth.

- **Learn from Criticism**: Use constructive criticism as a tool for improvement rather than viewing it as a personal attack.

- **Persevere in the face of setbacks**: See failures as a necessary part of the journey, a stepping stone rather than a stumbling block.

- **Celebrate effort, not just results**: By celebrating the effort put into a task, we reinforce the idea that growth comes from persistence and hard work.

Developing a Positive Attitude and Overcoming Negative Self-Talk

A positive attitude is not about ignoring life's challenges but about approaching them with optimism and proactive problem-solving. This positive outlook enables you to see opportunities where others see obstacles, helping you navigate through difficulties and bounce back from setbacks more swiftly.

Negative self-talk can be a substantial barrier to developing a positive attitude. Therefore, strategies for overcoming negative self-talk are vital. These include:

- **Recognize and acknowledge**: Be aware of your inner dialogue. Whenever you catch yourself engaging in negative self-talk, acknowledge it without judgment.

- **Challenge and Reframe**: Challenge negative thoughts. Is there evidence to support this thought? Is there another way to view this situation? Reframing involves seeing things from a different, more positive perspective.

- **Practice Affirmations**: Regular use of positive affirmations can help shift your inner dialogue to a more positive tone over time.

The Role of Self-Reflection and Self-Awareness in Mindset Shifts

Self-reflection and self-awareness are integral to shifting mindsets. They involve understanding your thoughts, emotions, and reactions, recognizing patterns in your behavior, and identifying areas for change. With self-reflection, you can challenge your old beliefs, discover new perspectives, and nurture a mindset that aligns with your goals. Tools for self-reflection can include journaling, meditation, and mindfulness practices.

The Role of Gratitude in Mindset Shifts

Gratitude plays a pivotal role in mindset shifts. It allows you to focus on what is going well, recognize the good in your life, and foster a more positive outlook. The practice of gratitude has been linked with increased happiness, reduced depression, and improved resilience. Simple strategies include keeping a gratitude journal, expressing thanks to others, and regularly reflecting on things you appreciate.

Practice gratitude daily. Write down things you're grateful for, express thanks to others, and take time each day to appreciate what you have. This habit can help foster a more positive, resilient mindset.

In conclusion, a mindset shift isn't an overnight event. It is a gradual process that requires conscious effort and practice. It involves challenging old beliefs and embracing new ways of thinking. This journey may seem arduous, but the benefits are immense. A shift in mindset can profoundly transform our lives, making us more resilient, adaptable, and open to growth. It lays the foundation for mental toughness, propelling us to overcome obstacles, strive towards our goals, and embrace the challenges life throws at us with grace and grit.

Implementing and Sustaining the Mindset Shift

Maintaining a growth mindset and sustaining a mindset shift take conscious, deliberate action. Here are some practical strategies:

1. **Continued Self-Reflection**: Regular self-reflection enables us to stay aware of our thoughts and behaviors, helping us to identify when we are slipping back into fixed mindset patterns.

2. **Mindful Living**: Practice being present in the moment. This helps us react to situations more thoughtfully and prevents us from falling into reactive, fixed-mindset behaviors.

3. **Consistent Learning**: Continue learning and pushing your boundaries. Embrace lifelong learning as a core part of your mindset.

4. **Support Network**: Surround yourself with positive, supportive individuals who encourage your growth mindset. Their support can help reinforce your mindset shift and keep you motivated.

5. **Gratitude Journaling**: Maintain a daily gratitude journal. This practice trains your mind to seek out the positive and fosters a positive, growth-oriented mindset.

Remember, the journey to a mindset shift is a marathon, not a sprint. Be patient with yourself, celebrate your progress, and remember that every step, no matter how small, brings you closer to becoming mentally tougher.

By mastering the art of mindset shift, you not only pave the way for developing mental toughness, but also set the stage for a life of continuous learning, growth, and resilience. The journey might seem challenging, but remember that growth comes through effort and consistency. Embrace the challenge, persist through the obstacles, and keep moving forward. Your journey towards a more resilient, mentally tough self begins with a shift in mindset. Let's embrace this journey together.

Chapter 9: Personal Stories

Personal stories are incredibly powerful. They put a face to the concepts and principles we've been discussing throughout this book. They show how real people, just like you and me, can apply the principles of mental toughness, overcome personal challenges, develop resilience, achieve goals, and overcome obstacles. In this chapter, we will explore some inspiring stories that will resonate with you, motivate you, and, above all, show you that mental toughness is indeed attainable.

This chapter presents inspiring stories of individuals who have exemplified mental toughness in their lives, showing how the concepts discussed in this book can be applied in practical, real-world situations.

Mental Toughness Mindset

Story: The Turnaround of David Atwood

David Atwood was on the edge of despair when his first venture, a tech startup, failed. The product didn't meet market demands, and the investors pulled out, leaving him drowning in debt and his confidence shattered. For a while, David wallowed in self-pity, feeling the sting of failure acutely.

But David, instead of wallowing for too long, chose to shift his mindset. He started seeing failure not as a dead-end, but as a detour. He accepted the failure, analyzed what went wrong, and began seeing the situation as a valuable learning experience rather than a personal defeat. This change in mindset marked the beginning of David's journey toward mental toughness.

Through his newfound perspective, David returned to the drawing board, this time focusing on market needs rather than personal interests. He launched a new venture in digital marketing, an area he recognized as a growing field. Today, David runs a successful digital marketing agency and mentors other aspiring entrepreneurs, instilling in them the power of a mentally tough mindset.

- **Reflection Prompts:** Have you ever faced a failure that left you feeling hopeless? How did you respond?

_____

_____

_____

_____

_____

_____

_____

_____

_____

_____

_____

_____

_____

- **Action Steps:** Reflect on a past failure. What did you learn from it? How can you apply those lessons to future challenges?

_____

_____

_____

_____

_____

_____

_____

_____

_____

_____

_____

_____

_____

_____

- **Invitation for Sharing: Do you have a story about adopting a mentally tough mindset? We'd love to hear it! Share your story on our dedicated platform and inspire others with it.**

- **Key Takeaways: Failure can be a valuable teacher. Embracing a mentally tough mindset allows us to learn from our mistakes and use them as stepping stones to success.**

Physical fitness and mental toughness

Story: Lara's Transformation through Endurance Running

Lara was a desk-bound software engineer with little physical activity in her routine. After a health scare and a stern warning from her doctor, Lara realized she needed to change. Given her sedentary lifestyle, she initially found the prospect of exercise intimidating. But as she committed to a training regime to prepare for a marathon, something unexpected happened.

The discipline, the persistence, and the regular confrontation with physical discomfort began transforming not just her body but her mind. She began to notice that the resilience she was building through her physical fitness regimen was spilling over into other areas of her life. She found herself better able to handle workplace stress, more patient with solving complex software problems, and generally more positive.

Completing her first marathon was a triumph for Lara and a testament to the transformation of her body and mind. Today, Lara continues to be an avid runner, crediting her physical fitness journey for her enhanced mental toughness.

- **Reflection Prompts: Have you ever challenged yourself physically in a way that resulted in mental growth? How did this challenge transform your mindset?**

_____

_____

_____

_____

_____

_____

_____

_____

_____

_____

_____

_____

_____

_____

_____

_____

- **Invitation for Sharing:** Do you have a story about how physical fitness contributed to your mental toughness? We'd love to hear about your journey. Share your experiences and insights on our dedicated platform, and inspire others with your story.

- **Key takeaways:** Physical fitness is not just about improving our bodies. The discipline, dedication, and resilience required for physical training can be a powerful mechanism for building mental toughness.

- **Action Steps:** Identify one physical activity that you can commit to regularly. Start small if necessary, and gradually increase the intensity or duration. Pay attention to how this commitment influences your mindset and resilience.

Mental Fitness and the 75-Day Program

Story: Andrea's Journey through the 75-Day Challenge

Andrea, a single mother working two jobs, was always stressed and overworked. Feeling overwhelmed and under constant pressure, she came across the 75-Day Mental Toughness Challenge and decided to give it a shot.

With mindfulness exercises, cognitive workouts, and meditation being integral parts of the program, Andrea initially found it challenging to fit these into her busy schedule. However, with consistent effort, she started seeing a shift. She found herself less agitated, more focused, and overall more resilient towards daily pressures. She began to feel less and less of the constant mental fatigue she had been experiencing.

The program's impact was transformative for Andrea. By Day 75, not only had she developed a robust routine for mental fitness, but she had also gained a significant improvement in her overall well-being and the ability to handle her demanding lifestyle effectively.

The stories of David, Lara, and Andrea are inspiring examples of individuals who have demonstrated mental toughness in the face of adversity. In the chapters to follow, we will delve into more real-life stories that touch on aspects of goal setting, accountability, overcoming obstacles, developing resilience, and the mindset shift. These narratives will provide a tangible perspective on the strategies and concepts we've been exploring throughout this book.

- **Reflection Prompts: Have you ever faced a situation where you felt overwhelmed by stress? How did you cope with it? Can you envision incorporating a mental fitness program into your routine?**

_____

_____

_____

_____

_____

_____

_____

_____

_____

_____

_____

_____

_____

_____

_____

_____

- **Invitation for Sharing: Have you embarked on a mental fitness program or taken steps to enhance your mental resilience? We'd love to hear about your journey! Share your experiences and insights on our dedicated platform, and inspire others with your story.**

- **Key Takeaways: Regular mental fitness exercises, much like physical workouts, can greatly enhance our mental resilience and ability to handle stress. A systematic program like the 75-Day Challenge can offer a structured approach to developing mental toughness.**

- **Action Steps: Begin with a simple mindfulness exercise today. It could be as easy as spending five minutes in silence, focusing on your breath. Consider committing to a structured program like the 75-Day Challenge to enhance your mental fitness.**

Goal Setting

Story: Victor's Ascent to the Peak

Victor was a young man from a small town with dreams bigger than his circumstances. His ambition was to climb Mount Everest, a lofty goal that seemed impossible to most people in his community. Victor, however, was undeterred.

He began by setting smaller, more achievable goals, like climbing local hills, and then graduated to higher altitudes over time. Each small victory was a confidence booster, and each setback was a learning experience. His journey was not smooth, but his clear vision of the end goal kept him motivated.

Eventually, after years of systematic goal-setting and diligent preparation, Victor stood atop Mount Everest. His story is a testament to the power of setting clear, tangible goals and the role they play in fostering mental toughness.

- *Reflection Prompts:* **Think of a time you set a goal for yourself. What steps did you take to achieve it? Did you face any setbacks? How did you overcome them?**

_____

_____

_____

_____

_____

_____

_____

_____

_____

_____

_____

_____

_____

_____

_____

- *Invitation for Sharing:* How has goal-setting played a role in your journey towards mental toughness? We'd love to hear about your experiences on our platform.

- Key Takeaways: Setting clear, tangible goals is a crucial step in developing mental toughness. By breaking down a larger goal into smaller, manageable tasks, we can maintain our motivation and track our progress effectively.

- Action Steps: Identify a goal you'd like to achieve. Break it down into smaller tasks that can be achieved in the short term. Remember to celebrate your victories, no matter how small, and learn from any setbacks.

Accountability

Story: Nina's Path to Financial Independence

Nina was a college graduate drowning in student loan debt. She felt out of control and helpless. Then she decided to take charge and hold herself accountable for her financial situation.

Nina took on a second job and cut back on non-essential expenses. She tracked every penny she spent and made sure she made her loan payments on time. It was tough, but Nina was tougher. Her determination to be accountable for her decisions helped her become debt-free within five years.

Today, Nina is financially independent and runs a personal finance blog to help others struggling with debt. Her story underscores the importance of accountability in fostering mental toughness and achieving our goals.

- *Reflection Prompts:* **Can you recall a time when you felt overwhelmed by a situation?**

How did you respond? How could taking accountability have changed the outcome?

_____

_____

_____

_____

_____

_____

_____

_____

_____

_____

_____

_____

_____

- *Invitation for Sharing:* Have you experienced a situation where taking accountability led to a positive change? We'd love to hear your story on our platform.

- *Action Steps:* Identify an area of your life where you would like to have more control. What steps can you take to hold yourself accountable?

_____

_____

_____

_____

_____

_____

_____

_____

_____

_____

_____

_____

_____

_____

_____

- *Key Takeaways:* Accountability is a crucial aspect of mental toughness. Taking responsibility for our decisions empowers us to change our circumstances.

Overcoming Obstacles

Story: Ahmed's Journey to Education

Ahmed, a refugee, faced numerous obstacles in his pursuit of education. Despite the language barrier, financial difficulties, and societal resistance, Ahmed refused to let these hurdles deter him from his goal.

He took language classes, worked part-time jobs, and applied for every possible scholarship. His journey was marked by perseverance and an unwavering belief in the power of education. Ahmed is a university graduate and works as an advocate for refugee education rights.

His story serves as a powerful reminder that no obstacle is too great when met with determination and mental toughness.

- *Reflection Prompts:* **Have you ever faced seemingly insurmountable obstacles in your path? How did you respond? What** resources did you utilize to overcome these challenges?

_____

_____

_____

_____

_____

_____

_____

_____

_____

_____

_____

- *Invitation for Sharing:* We invite you to share your personal stories of overcoming obstacles. Your experiences can inspire and encourage others who may be facing similar challenges. Please share your story on our dedicated platform.

- *Key Takeaways:* Obstacles are inevitable in any journey, but they can be overcome with determination and the right strategies. Ahmed's story demonstrates that no obstacle is too great when met with perseverance and a mentally tough mindset.

- *Action Steps:*

- Identify an obstacle in your life.
- Brainstorm potential solutions or strategies to overcome this obstacle.
- Take one small step towards implementing these strategies.

Developing Resilience

Story: Mia's Return to the Stage

Mia, a professional ballet dancer, faced a major setback when she was injured during a performance, leading to a prolonged recovery period. This could have ended her career, but Mia chose to view it differently.

During her recovery, Mia focused on physical therapy, mental health, and slowly rebuilding her strength. She chose to accept her situation, adapt to her limitations, and patiently work towards recovery, showing remarkable resilience.

After a year, Mia returned to the stage with a performance even more breathtaking than before. Her story is a beautiful testament to the power of resilience and mental toughness in overcoming life's unexpected challenges.

- *Reflection Prompts:* **Can you recall a time when you faced a setback that felt like the end of your world? How did you respond?**

_____

_____

_____

_____

_____

_____

_____

_____

_____

_____

_____

_____

_____

_____

_____

- **How does Mia's story resonate with your experiences?**

_____

_____

_____

_____

_____

_____

_____

_____

_____

_____

_____

_____

_____

_____

_____

- *Invitation for Sharing:* Has there been a time when resilience has helped you overcome a major obstacle in your life? How did you grow from the experience? We would love to hear about your journey. Share your story with us on our dedicated platform. Your story could inspire others to foster resilience in their own lives.

- *Action Steps:* Reflect on a setback you've experienced. How did you handle it? How could you have handled it better?

_____

_____

_____

_____

_____

_____

_____

_____

_____

_____

_____

_____

_____

_____

_____

- Practice resilience by setting small challenges for yourself and overcoming them. Each small victory will build your resilience for larger challenges.

- *Key Takeaways:*

✛ Resilience is about accepting our circumstances, adapting to changes, and persisting in the face of adversity.

✛ Developing resilience is a crucial aspect of mental toughness. It enables us to recover from setbacks and come back even stronger.

Mindset Shift

Story: Jake's Transformation from a Pessimist to an Optimist

Jake was a chronic pessimist. He always expected the worst, which held him back in his career and personal life. One day, Jake realized how this mindset was holding him back, and he decided to change.

He started by consciously recognizing his negative thought patterns. Each time a pessimistic thought entered his mind, he challenged it with a positive one. It was a tough and slow process, but over time, Jake's mindset began to shift.

Today, Jake is a transformed man. His optimistic outlook has opened new opportunities in his life, proving that shifting one's mindset is a crucial step towards developing mental toughness.

Each of these stories illustrates how real people have applied the principles and strategies discussed in this book, demonstrating that developing mental toughness is a feasible and worthwhile endeavor for everyone.

- *Reflection Prompts:* **Do you identify with Jake's story? Are there areas in your life where you tend to lean towards pessimism? How has this affected your life?**

_____

_____

_____

_____

_____

_____

_____

_____

_____

_____

_____

_____

_____

_____

_____

_____

_____

_____

_____

- *Invitation for Sharing:* Have you successfully shifted from a pessimistic to an optimistic mindset? How did it impact your life? We invite you to share your story on our dedicated platform. Your journey can serve as an inspiration to others working towards a similar transformation.

- *Key Takeaways:* Recognizing and challenging negative thought patterns is the first step towards developing a positive mindset. This shift in mindset can dramatically influence our resilience, motivation, and overall success in life.

- *Action Steps:* Identify a particular area of your life where you notice negative thinking. Each time a negative thought arises, challenge it with a positive one. Keep a journal to track your progress.

Conclusion

As we conclude this journey through "Developing Mental Toughness: A 75-Day Challenge", let's take a moment to reflect on the crucial insights we've explored.

We delved into the importance of fostering a mental toughness mindset, a fundamental first step in facing challenges with courage and resilience. We saw how physical fitness contributes to mental toughness, demonstrating the intricate connection between our body and mind. Our exploration of the 75-Day Program emphasized the role of mental fitness in cultivating our cognitive abilities and emotional resilience.

We also discussed the power of setting tangible, achievable goals and how the journey towards these goals instills mental toughness. The principles of accountability showed us that owning our decisions, successes, and failures is integral to our growth and resilience.

By examining the process of overcoming obstacles, we understood that every hurdle presents an opportunity for growth and learning. Similarly, developing resilience taught us the value of bouncing back from adversity, while a shift in mindset can profoundly influence our perception of life's challenges.

While the 75-day program provides a robust framework for developing mental toughness, the real journey continues beyond the completion of this program. Every day presents new challenges and opportunities for growth. Mental toughness is not a destination but an ongoing journey. Remember, the skills and habits you have cultivated throughout this challenge are tools that you can continually utilize.

As you move forward, remember the personal stories shared in this book. These stories are proof that ordinary individuals, just like you, can cultivate extraordinary mental toughness. Draw inspiration from them and remind yourself of your potential.

Lastly, remember that you are not alone in your journey. Join the community of people dedicated to improving their mental toughness. Share your experiences, learn from others, and grow together.

Thank you for embarking on this 75-day challenge. Your commitment to developing mental toughness is commendable. Keep pushing your boundaries, stay resilient during adversity, hold yourself accountable, and continue to grow stronger mentally every day.

Remember, the only real limit to your abilities is the one you set for yourself. So keep challenging yourself, maintain your mental fitness, and continue this journey of mental toughness beyond these 75 days and into the rest of your life. Good luck, and stay mentally tough!

Printed in the USA
CPSIA information can be obtained
at www.ICGtesting.com
LVHW021620301023
762577LV00013B/166